Ripa Chakraborty, RDN (UK), BDS, MSc (Dental Public Health), is a UK-registered dental nurse with professional experience in primary dental care and a strong academic background in public health. Her work focuses on oral health promotion, prevention-focused service delivery, and the evolving role of dental nurses within multidisciplinary dental teams.

She holds a Bachelor of Dental Surgery and a master's degree in dental public health and has a particular interest in addressing oral health inequalities affecting children and underserved populations. Her research explores how workforce development, education, and policy can strengthen preventive care in general dental practice.

Ripa is committed to evidence-informed practice and translational research that supports sustainable, equitable oral healthcare systems.

AF689100

Preface

Dental caries remains one of the most common yet preventable chronic conditions affecting children worldwide. Despite significant advances in preventive dentistry, oral health inequalities continue to persist across and within countries, disproportionately affecting children from socioeconomically disadvantaged backgrounds. These inequalities highlight the need for practical, accessible, and prevention-focused models of care within everyday dental practice.

In recent years, increasing attention has been paid to the role of skill mix and team-based approaches in dentistry. Dental nurses, who frequently serve as a consistent point of contact for children and families within general dental practices, are uniquely positioned to support oral health promotion and disease prevention. However, despite their potential, the preventive roles of dental nurses remain underutilised, inconsistently defined, and unevenly implemented across different healthcare systems.

This book is intended for dental nurses, dental care professionals, educators, researchers, policymakers, and practitioners interested in prevention-focused dentistry. This book presents a scoping review of global evidence examining the roles of dental nurses in delivering oral health promotion activities to prevent dental caries in children in general dental practice settings. By systematically mapping existing research, this work seeks to clarify the nature and scope of dental nurse-led preventive activities, identify facilitators and barriers to their implementation, and highlight gaps in the current evidence base.

The aims of this book are threefold. First, it aims to provide a clear, accessible synthesis of existing evidence for students, educators, and researchers interested in dental public health and workforce development. Second, it aims to inform dental practitioners, policymakers, and commissioners about the potential contribution of dental nurses to prevention-led models of care. Finally, it seeks to identify priorities for future research, policy development, and training to strengthen dental nurses' roles in improving children's oral health outcomes.

By focusing on general dental practices—the primary setting for dental care in many countries—this book situates prevention within real-world clinical contexts. It is hoped that this work will contribute to ongoing discussions around workforce optimisation, preventive dentistry, and the future direction of child oral health services.

Acknowledgements

I would like to express my sincere gratitude to all who supported and encouraged me throughout the development of this work. My deepest thanks go to **Dr Vanessa Muirhead**, Professor and Head of Dental Public Health Faculty, whose academic guidance, expertise, and constructive feedback were invaluable in shaping the direction and quality of this review. I would also like to acknowledge the contributions of academic librarians and educators who guided the evidence synthesis and research methodology, thereby strengthening the rigour of this work.

On a personal note, I extend heartfelt thanks to my father, Dr Ram Kamal Chakraborty; my mother, Bina Chakraborty; my husband, Ranjan Chakraborty; and my two sons, Avash Chakraborty and Avirup Chakraborty, for their patience, encouragement, and unwavering support throughout this journey. Their belief in my aspirations made completing this work possible.

Finally, I am grateful to colleagues and peers whose discussions and shared perspectives enriched my understanding of dental public health and the evolving role of dental nurses in preventive care.

Abstract

Background:

Dental caries remains one of the most prevalent chronic conditions affecting children globally, despite being largely preventable. Persistent socioeconomic inequalities, limited access to preventive services, and inconsistent utilisation of the dental workforce continue to contribute to disease burden. Dental nurses are increasingly recognised as key contributors to oral health promotion within general dental practice; however, evidence regarding their specific roles and effectiveness in caries prevention remains fragmented and inconsistently reported.

Aim:

This scoping review aimed to systematically map and synthesise global evidence on the roles of dental nurses in promoting oral health and preventing dental caries among children aged 0–18 years within general dental practice settings.

Methods:

A scoping review was conducted in accordance with the Joanna Briggs Institute (JBI) methodology and guided by the Population–Concept–Context (PCC) framework. A comprehensive search of five electronic databases and relevant grey literature was undertaken. Eligible studies included those reporting dental nurse–led or dental nurse–supported preventive interventions targeting paediatric dental caries. Data were extracted using a structured charting tool and analysed using narrative synthesis.

Results:
Ten studies met the inclusion criteria, with the majority originating from high-income countries, particularly the United Kingdom. Dental nurses were involved in a range of preventive activities, most commonly fluoride varnish application, oral health education, and supervised tooth brushing. One randomised controlled trial demonstrated a reduction in caries incidence following a dental nurse–led intervention, while the remaining studies employed observational or descriptive designs. Identified barriers included limited training opportunities, restrictive workforce policies, unclear role delineation, and inconsistent integration within dental teams. Facilitators included structured education and training programmes, supportive organisational frameworks, and multidisciplinary collaboration.

Conclusion:
The findings indicate that dental nurses have the potential to play a meaningful role in preventing dental caries in children within general dental practice settings. However, the current evidence base is limited by methodological weaknesses, geographic concentration, and a lack of long-term outcome evaluation. Strengthening policy support, standardising training pathways, and expanding high-quality research are essential to optimise dental nurses' contributions to preventive oral healthcare and reduce oral health inequalities among children.

Author's Note:

This book is written for dental nurses, dental care professionals, dental students, educators, researchers, general dental practitioners, practice managers, policymakers, commissioners, and public health professionals who share an interest in oral health promotion, preventive dentistry, and the effective development of the dental workforce. It is intended to serve as both an academic resource and a practical reference for those seeking to improve oral health outcomes for children in general dental practice.

Grounded in contemporary research and informed by current professional and policy contexts, this work brings together evidence on the role of dental nurses in supporting preventive oral health initiatives. It seeks to present a clear, structured synthesis of existing knowledge while highlighting how dental nurses contribute meaningfully to the delivery of preventive care, patient education, and broader public health objectives. Particular attention is given to the integration of dental nurses within multidisciplinary dental teams and how their skills can support equitable, efficient, and prevention-focused models of care.

While firmly rooted in academic scholarship, this book has been written with accessibility in mind. Complex concepts are presented clearly and practically to ensure relevance for practitioners, educators, service planners, and decision-makers. The intention of development and evidence-informed practice encourages reflective professional development and contributes to informed discussions around workforce utilisation and service design within dentistry.

Looking forward, this work aims to contribute to ongoing dialogue and future development in preventive oral healthcare. By highlighting existing practices, emerging opportunities, and areas for strategic growth, it seeks to support continued innovation, policy development, and research that strengthen dental nurses' roles in improving oral health outcomes for children. Ultimately, the book aspires to support a more preventive, collaborative, and sustainable approach to dental care that benefits patients, professionals, and health systems alike.

Table of Contents

List of Figures, Charts, and Tables

List of Abbreviations

Abbreviation	Full Form
OHP	Oral Health Promotion
ECC	Early Childhood Caries
NHS	National Health Service
WHO	World Health Organisation
GDC	General Dental Council
JBI	Joanna Briggs Institute
PRISMA-ScR	Preferred Reporting Items for Systematic Reviews and Meta-Analyses – Scoping Review
RCT	Randomised Controlled Trial

DMFT/dmft	Decayed, Missing and Filled Teeth (Index)
PICO/PCC	Population, Intervention, Comparison, Outcome / Population, Concept, Context
OHE	Oral Health Education
CPD	Continuing Professional Development
UK	United Kingdom
UDC	Urgent Dental Care
QIP	Quality Improvement Project
PDF	Portable Document Format
BPE	Basic Periodontal Examination

CHAPTER 1: INTRODUCTION

1.1 Background and Global Burden:

Dental caries, also known as tooth decay, is the most widespread non-communicable disease (NCD) globally, particularly affecting children at an alarming rate, despite being largely preventable, according to the World Health Organisation (WHO, 2017). This persistent and complex condition results from a myriad of influences, including dietary choices, oral hygiene practices, fluoride exposure, and broader social determinants such as socioeconomic status and access to healthcare.

The 2019 Global Burden of Disease Study revealed a staggering statistic: untreated dental caries in primary teeth affects over 620 million children worldwide, ranking it among the top ten most prevalent health issues globally (WHO, 2023). This highlights the urgent need for ongoing attention to oral health, particularly among vulnerable populations.

In high-income countries, efforts such as community-based water fluoridation programs, widespread oral health promotion initiatives, and accessible preventive dental services have led to significant improvements in dental health outcomes. However, these advances have not been uniformly experienced; pronounced disparities in oral health outcomes persist within and across countries. According to studies by Sheiham (2006) and Watt and Sheiham (2012), these inequalities underscore the importance of addressing both individual and systemic factors that contribute to the persistence of dental caries, particularly among children who may lack access to essential oral health resources.

Figure 1 presents a detailed bar chart showing a significant decline in dental caries prevalence as income levels increase across various countries. The data are particularly striking in low- and middle-income nations, where dental caries rates are alarmingly high. For instance, Nigeria has an astounding dental caries rate of 85%, while India follows closely with 80%. In comparison, upper-middle-income countries such as Egypt exhibit more moderate rates, with approximately 65% of the population affected by dental caries.

In stark contrast, high-income countries tend to experience significantly lower rates of dental caries. For example, the prevalence in the United Kingdom is around 50%, and Australia reports an even lower rate of 35%. This observable trend highlights a crucial correlation: as national income and access to quality dental care improve, the rates of dental caries decline correspondingly. This situation highlights the urgent need to implement effective oral health promotion strategies tailored to the diverse needs of communities at both global and local levels. Emphasising oral health education, access to preventive services, and affordable dental care will be essential in addressing these disparities.

Figure 1. Country-level prevalence of dental caries in children. Data Source: (WHO, 2017; Global Burden of Disease Study, 2019).

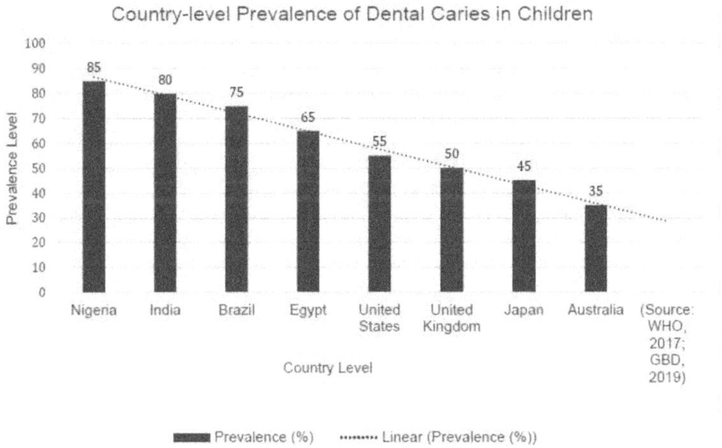

As illustrated, the prevalence of childhood dental caries varies significantly worldwide, with notably higher rates observed in lower- and middle-income countries (WHO, 2017; GBD, 2019). This stark disparity is often linked to systemic social inequalities, limited oral health literacy, and a lack of integration of oral health services into primary healthcare systems. While high-income countries, such as the United Kingdom, Sweden, and Australia, have seen improvements in oral health outcomes, significant disparities remain, particularly among ethnic minorities and low-income families (Watt & Sheiham, 2012).

Recognising the need for global action, the WHO Global Oral Health Action Plan 2023–2030 urges all countries to incorporate oral health into universal health coverage. It also calls for the mobilisation of mid-level oral health workers, such as dental nurses, to take active roles in preventing oral diseases (WHO, 2023).

Figure 2: The WHO Global Oral Health Action Plan 2023–2030 (Source: WHO.int, 2024)

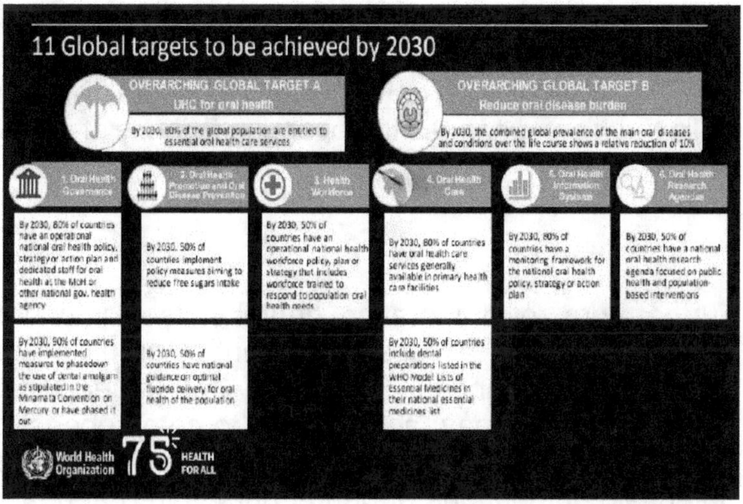

Oral health promotion plays a crucial role in preventing dental caries, one of the most prevalent oral health issues. Historically, the responsibility for this vital aspect of dental care has rested primarily with dentists and dental hygienists. However, there is growing recognition of the importance of a more collaborative approach involving the entire dental team. This is particularly true for dental nurses, especially those who have received specialised training to perform extended duties.

In the United Kingdom, dental nurses registered with the General Dental Council (GDC) are authorised to engage in various preventive activities, provided they work under appropriate supervision. These activities encompass a range of essential services, including giving oral hygiene instructions to improve patient practices, applying fluoride varnish to strengthen enamel and reduce caries risk, and offering dietary advice tailored to promote better oral health. This inclusive model not only leverages dental nurses' skills but also enhances the overall efficiency of dental practices.

Furthermore, by integrating dental nurses into oral health promotion, access to preventive care can be significantly enhanced, particularly for underserved populations that may face barriers to comprehensive dental services. Despite these advantages, the potential contributions of dental nurses in oral health promotion remain largely untapped in many areas. This underutilization can be attributed to various systemic challenges and workforce constraints that limit their engagement in preventive care initiatives. These factors underscore the need for ongoing efforts to better integrate dental nurses into the broader healthcare team, ensuring that their valuable skills are fully leveraged for the benefit of patients and communities alike.

1.2 The UK Context and Oral Health Inequalities

In the United Kingdom, the overall oral health of children has shown notable improvements in recent years; however, significant health inequalities persist, posing a major challenge. According to a report by Public Health England (PHE, 2022), approximately 23.7% of five-year-old children in England have experienced dental decay. This statistic highlights a pressing public health concern, particularly given the significant disparities across geographic regions and socioeconomic statuses.

The data reveal that children from the most deprived communities are disproportionately affected by dental health issues, showing a troubling trend where they are three times more likely to suffer from caries compared to their counterparts in more affluent areas (PHE, 2022). For instance, recent findings indicate that 34.3% of five-year-olds in the most deprived quintile experience dental caries, in stark contrast to only 13.6% in the least deprived quintile (PHE, 2022).

This disparity highlights not only differences in access to dental care and oral hygiene education but also raises broader questions about the social determinants of health. Factors such as income, education, and access to health services play a pivotal role in these inequalities. Efforts to bridge this gap are essential to ensure that all children, regardless of their socioeconomic background, have the opportunity to achieve optimal oral health and overall well-being. Addressing these issues requires targeted interventions and policies that focus on equitable access to dental care and preventive education tailored to the needs of disadvantaged communities.

Table 1: Prevalence and Severity of Dental Caries Among 5-Year-Olds in England by Deprivation Quintile (PHE,2022).

Deprivation Quintile (IMD)	% with Dental Caries	Mean dmft Score	% with Untreated Decay
Quintile 1 (Most Deprived)	34.3%	1.55	25.0%
Quintile 2	28.1%	1.20	19.6%
Quintile 3	22.7%	0.90	15.0%
Quintile 4	18.9%	0.68	11.3%
Quintile 5 (Least Deprived)	13.6%	0.48	8.5%

The disparities in dental health outcomes are influenced by a complex interplay of factors, including parents' educational attainment, household income, family members' dietary choices, and the availability and accessibility of preventive dental care services (Watt & Sheiham, 2012). Recognising the significance of these determinants, dental public health policies increasingly emphasise early intervention strategies. Moreover, they advocate for collaborative, team-based approaches to preventive care within general dental practices. This shift aims to create more comprehensive care frameworks that address immediate dental issues and promote long-term oral health through education and access to preventive services.

1.3 General Dental Practices and Oral Health Promotion

General dental practices function as a foundational entry point for children and families seeking dental care, playing a crucial role in their oral health journey. In addition to providing essential clinical treatments, these practices also offer valuable opportunities to deliver targeted oral health education and preventive measures. The Delivering Better Oral Health toolkit (DBOH v4) champions a collaborative, team-oriented approach to prevention, offering comprehensive guidance on key aspects such as effective toothbrushing techniques, nutritional choices that support dental health, the application of fluoride varnish, and structured recall scheduling to ensure ongoing care (OHID, 2021). This model empowers all dental professionals—dentists, hygienists, and dental nurses alike—to actively participate in health education and provide behavioural support to foster positive oral health habits in their young patients and their families.

The effectiveness of preventive strategies in general practice is closely tied to the involvement of the broader dental team. Dental nurses, in particular, are ideally positioned to deliver consistent, child-friendly oral health messages. They can provide practical demonstrations and advice during routine appointments. Because they are familiar with patients and their families and are consistently present during care pathways, dental nurses can effectively reinforce preventive guidance in an accessible and supportive way (Anderson et al., 2020).

1.4 Expanding Roles of Dental Nurses in Oral Health Promotion

In recent years, the role of dental nurses in the UK has undergone significant advancements, reflecting changes in both healthcare practices and patient needs. As outlined by the General Dental Council (GDC) in 2023, dental nurses who undergo specialised training are now authorised to perform additional responsibilities, such as applying fluoride varnish, conducting oral health education sessions, and facilitating behaviour change interventions, all under appropriate supervision. This expansion of duties has become increasingly promoted within NHS policies and training guidelines, particularly as a response to ongoing workforce shortages and the growing need for preventive dental care services.

Evidence from successful initiatives, such as Childsmile in Scotland, illustrates the substantial benefits of involving dental nurses in community-based programs. These programs include supervised toothbrushing sessions in schools to instil proper oral hygiene habits in children, as well as the application of fluoride varnish to protect against tooth decay.

Research by Kidd et al. (2020) demonstrates that these collaborative efforts improve oral health outcomes among young participants.

Despite these advancements, much of the existing literature tends either to generalise the responsibilities of dental nurses by conflating them with those of other oral health professionals or to fall short of providing a thorough evaluation of the specific outcomes of interventions led by dental nurses. As healthcare systems increasingly transition towards prevention-focused models, it becomes crucial to define clearly the scope of practice for dental nurses and to assess the effectiveness of dental nurse-led oral health programs in achieving positive health outcomes.

Across the globe, the role of dental nurses in promoting oral health presents a fascinating tapestry of diversity and disparity. In certain countries, their responsibilities are primarily confined to providing chairside assistance and ensuring the meticulous sterilisation of instruments, often relegated to the background of the dental practice. Conversely, in other regions, dental nurses are empowered with extensive training and official authorisation to spearhead vibrant oral health initiatives in schools and communities, becoming champions of dental education and oral health. This striking variation in training, regulation, and the scope of practice creates significant challenges when evaluating the overall influence of dental nurses on children's oral health outcomes, hindering a comprehensive picture of their global impact.

Although there is increasing awareness of the vital role dental nurses play, there is still insufficient consolidated evidence on how they help reduce caries in children, especially in general dental practices. These practices are the primary setting for dental care in many countries. Figure 3 illustrates how dental nurses work alongside dentists and hygienists in general practice, highlighting their specific contributions to prevention.

Figure 3: Roles of Dental Team Members in Prevention Adapted from GDC (2023) and OHID (2021).

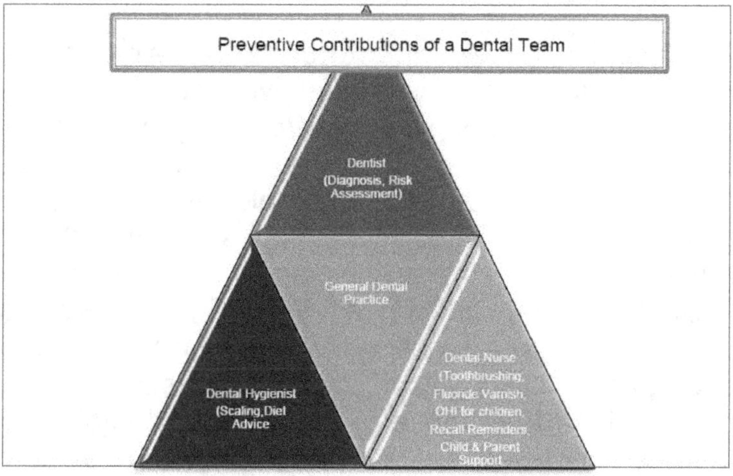

These professionals often develop close rapport with families, especially children, which enables them to reinforce oral health advice in a more engaging and supportive manner. Their participation is crucial in reaching underserved populations and ensuring continuity of care.

1.5 The Research Gap and Rationale for Review

Despite national policies aimed at promoting skill mix within dental teams, a significant research gap persists in examining dental nurses' contributions to caries prevention among children in general dental practice. The majority of available studies focus on interventions in community or school environments or are found in grey literature, which often lacks methodological rigour and consistency. Additionally, comprehensive international comparative data on this topic are limited.

This scoping review aims to systematically map the global evidence on the preventive roles that dental nurses play in caring for children in general dental practices. The review seeks to explore the various interventions dental nurses implement to prevent tooth decay, the specific training and support they receive to perform these roles, and the challenges and facilitators that influence their involvement in preventive care. Existing research often fails to adequately distinguish dental nurses' unique contributions from those of the broader dental team, thereby complicating our understanding of their specific responsibilities and impacts (Anderson et al., 2020).

ADDITIONALLY, SUBSTANTIAL VARIATIONS IN TRAINING, RESPONSIBILITIES, AND DEPLOYMENT OF DENTAL NURSES FURTHER COMPLICATE EFFORTS TO CLARIFY THEIR ROLES WITHIN DENTAL PRACTICES (GDC, 2023). THEREFORE, CONDUCTING A SCOPING REVIEW IS ESSENTIAL NOT ONLY TO IDENTIFY RESEARCH GAPS BUT ALSO TO INFORM FUTURE POLICY DEVELOPMENT AND BEST PRACTICES IN PEDIATRIC DENTAL CARE.

1.6 RESEARCH AIM, QUESTION, AND PCC FRAMEWORK

This study aims to systematically identify and map the oral health promotion activities that dental nurses provide to children in general dental practices. Specifically, it addresses the following research question:

Research Question:

- What is the global evidence for dental nurses (Population) providing oral health promotion activities (Concept) to prevent caries in children in dental practices (Context)?

The question is framed using the Population, Concept, and Context (PCC) structure recommended by the Joanna Briggs Institute (JBI) for scoping reviews:

- **Population:** Trained and registered dental nurses, including dental auxiliaries, dental assistants and Extended-duty dental nurses.
- **Concept:** Oral health promotion activities to prevent dental caries, such as toothbrushing advice, fluoride varnish applications, diet counselling, oral health education, and behavioural change interventions like motivational interviewing.
- **Context:** General dental practices (NHS or private) globally targeting children aged 0–18.

1.7 OBJECTIVES

The review objectives were as follows:

- To identify dental nurses' oral health promotion activities in different countries.
- To identify the groups of children dental nurses target in dental practices globally, including those from different socioeconomic backgrounds, age groups (e.g., those with early childhood caries), regular attenders, and high-risk children.
- To assess the outcomes measured in studies involving dental nurses, including clinical outcomes (e.g., reduction in caries incidence), patient-reported outcomes (e.g., changes in attitudes or behaviours), and intermediate outcomes (e.g., uptake of fluoride varnish or improved oral hygiene practices).
- To identify studies that assessed the effectiveness of dental nurse-led interventions in preventing dental caries in children within dental practices.

1.8 Significance of the Study

The findings of this scoping review will help map global practices, inform workforce planning, and guide policy and training. By identifying where dental nurses are most effectively used, this research aims to reduce oral health inequalities and support evidence-based care models in primary dental settings.

1.9 STRUCTURE OF THE DISSERTATION

This dissertation is structured into six chapters. Chapter 2 reviews the existing literature relevant to dental nurses' roles in oral health promotion. Chapter 3 describes the methodology of the scoping review, detailing the search strategy, inclusion criteria, and data extraction processes. Chapter 4 presents the results of the included studies (including PRISMA chart and evidence tables), and Chapter 5 discusses their findings and implications about existing policy, education, and practice. Chapter 6 concludes the study by providing recommendations and identifying areas for future research.

CHAPTER 2: LITERATURE REVIEW

2.1 BACKGROUND:

This chapter examines existing evidence on the role of dental nurses in promoting oral health (OHP), with a specific focus on preventing dental caries in children within general dental practices. It synthesises studies from both global and UK contexts, focusing on the evolution of the dental nurse's role and the enablers and barriers to effective implementation. Additionally, it identifies key gaps in research. This chapter lays the groundwork for the scoping review by providing the rationale and context for exploring prevention efforts led by dental nurses.

2.2 The Burden of Dental Caries in Children:

Dental caries is one of the most common chronic conditions affecting children worldwide. According to the World Health Organisation (WHO, 2017), between 60% and 90% of school-aged children are affected, especially in low- and middle-income countries. The Global Burden of Disease (GBD, 2019) identifies untreated dental caries in primary teeth as one of the top ten global health burdens for this age group.

In the UK, Public Health England (PHE, 2022) reports that 23.7% of five-year-old children in England experience dental decay. This prevalence increases to 34.3% among children in the most deprived socioeconomic quintiles. These statistics highlight a significant socioeconomic gradient in oral health outcomes, underscoring the need for community-based, accessible preventive interventions.

2.3 Oral Health Promotion and Prevention in Primary Care

Oral health promotion strategies within primary care include fluoride varnish application, oral hygiene instruction, diet counselling, and risk-based recall planning. Cooper et al. (2013) highlight that these interventions effectively reduce caries and engage families in the prevention process. The OHID's Delivering Better Oral Health (DBOH v4) toolkit outlines evidence-based prevention tailored for dental practices (OHID, 2021).

Repeated dental visits offer opportunities to reinforce healthy behaviours, especially for young children. However, these opportunities are often missed due to limited team engagement. Watt and Sheiham (2012) advocate for a team-based prevention model in which all members of the dental team, including nurses, contribute to health promotion.

2.4 The Role of Dental Nurses in Oral Health Promotion

The role of dental nurses in prevention has undergone significant evolution, particularly in the UK. The

General Dental Council (GDC) outlines a broad scope of practice for dental nurses, including oral health education, fluoride varnish application, and participation in preventive campaigns, provided they receive appropriate training (GDC, 2023). Dental nurses are also encouraged to undertake additional qualifications such as the NEBDN Certificate in Oral Health Education or Fluoride Application.

Several studies support the idea that dental nurses can be practical in delivering OHP. Anderson et al. (2020) found that dental nurses who engaged in brief interventions—such as fluoride varnish application and diet advice—during children's appointments helped reinforce preventive messages and improve parental compliance. Harris et al. (2012) similarly demonstrated the feasibility of including trained dental nurses in prevention-focused roles during recall appointments.

Several studies have explored the preventive roles of dental nurses, highlighting their involvement in fluoride varnish application, oral hygiene instruction, and patient education. Table 2 summarises key studies that examine the scope, interventions, and outcomes of dental nurses' participation in oral health promotion for children. These studies reflect the diversity of settings and methodologies used to evaluate their impact.

Table 2: Summary of Key Studies on Dental Nurses' Role in Oral Health Promotion in Children.

Author (Year)	Country	Study Design	Intervention/Focus	Key Findings
Harris et al. (2012)	UK	Randomised Control Trial	Fluoride varnish & dietary advice	Improved parental compliance, reduced risk factors
Cooper et al. (2013)	UK	Systematic Review	School-based and practice-based OHP	OHP is effective in changing behaviours
Anderson et al. (2020)	Australia	Qualitative study	Dental nurse-delivered OHE in clinics	High acceptability and trust among parents

Dental nurses are often trusted by families, particularly those who attend regularly, and their continuity of care makes them suitable messengers for health advice. However, most of the evidence in this area remains descriptive, focusing on feasibility and acceptability rather than long-term effectiveness. This limits the generalizability of findings.

2.5 Global Variation in Dental Nurse Roles

Internationally, the utilisation of dental nurses for health promotion varies widely. In high-income countries such as the UK, New Zealand, and Australia, dental nurses (or dental therapists) often receive formal training and are integrated into health promotion teams. However, in many low- and Middle-income countries, their roles are limited to chairside assistance or sterilisation, and they are seldom trained or authorised to deliver preventive care (Ribeiro et al., 2014).

In some contexts, particularly in Asia and Africa, oral health promotion is primarily carried out in community or school settings by outreach workers, and the role of dental nurses in general practice remains underdeveloped. This variability complicates global comparisons of effectiveness and underscores the need for greater clarity and standardisation.

2.6 Enablers and Barriers to Dental Nurse Involvement

Several enablers support dental nurses' involvement in oral health promotion. These include supportive practice environments (Anderson et al., 2020), structured team communication, access to continuing professional development CPD (GDC, 2023), and clear guidance from regulators and policy bodies (OHID, 2021). When dental nurses are confident and competent in delivering key messages, they can reduce the burden on dentists and contribute to more efficient, child-friendly care pathways.

However, several barriers remain. These include limited time during appointments, lack of funding or incentives for prevention, hierarchical team dynamics, and inconsistent implementation of training schemes

(Cooper et al., 2013). In many practices, dental nurses report feeling underprepared or undervalued in delivering health education due to inadequate supervision or organisational culture.

2.7 Gaps in Literature

Despite policy emphasis on prevention, empirical evidence on the direct impact of dental nurses in reducing dental caries remains sparse. Much of the literature consists of pilot studies, case reports, or grey literature, with few high-quality trials or outcome evaluations. Additionally, most research aggregates dental nurses' roles with those of other professionals, making it difficult to isolate their specific contributions.

There is also a lack of comparative international data. Most studies available originate in the UK, with limited input from other high- or low-income settings. Moreover, few studies have examined the cost-effectiveness or long-term outcomes of dental nurse-led OHP interventions in general dental practice.

2.8 Summary

The literature demonstrates that dental nurses play a promising role in promoting children's oral health, particularly in general dental practices. Their involvement in fluoride varnish, dietary counselling, and education aligns with national and international guidelines. However, the overall evidence base lacks high-quality trials, long-term data, and global representation. This scoping review addresses these gaps by systematically mapping current evidence and informing future practice and policy.

CHAPTER 3: METHODOLOGY

3.1 INTRODUCTION

This chapter outlines the methodological approach used to conduct a scoping review of the role of dental nurses in delivering oral health promotion (OHP) interventions to prevent dental caries in children within general dental practices. The review adhered to the Joanna Briggs Institute (JBI) guidelines for scoping reviews (Peters et al., 2020) and the PRISMA-ScR (Preferred Reporting Items for Systematic Reviews and Meta-Analyses extension for Scoping Reviews) checklist (Tricco et al., 2018).

The following sections detail the review design, eligibility criteria, search strategy, study selection process, and data extraction and synthesis procedures. All included studies were critically appraised using the relevant Joanna Briggs Institute (JBI) Critical Appraisal Checklists (JBI, 2024). The checklist employed corresponded to the specific study designs, including randomised controlled trials (RCTs), cross-sectional studies, qualitative studies, and quasi-experimental studies.

3.2 Study Design and Justification:

Given the broad nature of the research question and the diverse evidence base, a scoping review was selected as the most appropriate method. Unlike systematic reviews, scoping reviews are well-suited for examining emerging areas and heterogeneous studies where key concepts are not yet well-established (Munn et al., 2018). This design enabled a comprehensive exploration of the various roles dental nurses play in caries prevention, without requiring critical appraisal of the included studies.

3.3 PCC Framework and Review Question

The scoping review was meticulously organised using the JBI's Population–Concept–Context (PCC) framework, a tool designed to aid researchers in establishing precise eligibility criteria while effectively directing the search and synthesis of relevant literature. The primary review question was articulated as follows:

'What is the specific role of dental nurses in implementing oral health promotion interventions aimed at preventing dental caries among children in general dental practice settings?'

The Population segment of the review encompassed trained and registered dental nurses, including those with specialised skills, such as Extended Duties Dental Nurses (EDDNs). These practitioners are directly involved in delivering a range of interventions to pediatric patients, ensuring they are equipped to address children's unique dental needs.

The Concept dimension focused on a range of preventive oral health promotion activities pivotal to combating dental caries. This includes specific practices such as the application of fluoride varnish, which has been shown to reduce the incidence of caries significantly; oral health education (OHE) that empowers children and their families with knowledge about maintaining dental hygiene; supervised toothbrushing initiatives that encourage proper brushing techniques; motivational interviewing (MI) that fosters positive behavior change regarding oral health; and dietary counseling which informs families about nutritional choices that impact dental health.

The Context component defined the settings in which these interventions take place, specifically, general dental practices across various regions worldwide. This encompasses both the National Health Service (NHS) and private primary care settings, illustrating the broad applicability of dental nurses' roles across healthcare systems.

3.4 Definitions of Key Terms

In alignment with the review objectives, several key terms were defined.

Dental nurses are qualified and registered professionals who carry out clinical preventive activities under a dentist's supervision.

Children were defined as individuals aged 0 to 18 years, in accordance with the WHO and UN conventions. General dental practice encompassed primary care dental settings, rather than specialist paediatric, hospital-based, or purely community outreach programmes.

Dental caries was understood as a sugar-driven, biofilm-mediated disease characterised by enamel and dentine demineralisation.

Oral health promotion interventions included educational, behavioural, or clinical activities aimed at reducing caries risk or incidence.

3.5 Inclusion and Exclusion Criteria

3.5.1 Inclusion Criteria

Studies were included if they evaluated interventions delivered by dental nurses or EDDNs targeting children aged 0–18 years. Interventions had to be implemented within general dental practices, either public or private, and aimed to prevent or reduce dental caries. Eligible study designs included randomised controlled trials (RCTs), before–and–after studies, observational studies, cross-sectional surveys, programme evaluations, rapid reviews, and scoping reviews. Studies are needed to report outcomes related to caries incidence, oral health behaviours, knowledge, or service use, such as appointment attendance.

3.5.2 Exclusion Criteria

Studies were excluded if interventions were delivered solely by dentists, therapists, or hygienists, without dental nurse involvement. Articles focusing exclusively on adults or offered only in schools or community settings without a link to general dental practices were omitted. Editorials, letters, and studies lacking original data were also excluded. These criteria were applied at both the title/abstract and full-text screening stages.

3.6 Search Strategy

A comprehensive and systematic literature search was conducted across four prominent electronic databases—namely, PubMed, Scopus, Embase, and Web of Science—on June 15, 2025. The search strategy was meticulously crafted using the Population–Concept–Context (PCC) framework, as recommended by the Joanna Briggs Institute (Peters et al., 2020). This methodical approach employed Boolean operators and truncation to combine a tailored set of keywords with relevant Medical Subject Headings (MeSH) terms.

The primary objective of this extensive search was to identify and evaluate studies that specifically investigate the role of dental nurses in promoting oral health, with particular focus on their involvement in preventing dental caries among pediatric patients in general dental practice. To achieve this, the search strategy integrated keywords and MeSH terms such as “dental nurse,” “oral health promotion,” “fluoride varnish application,” “toothbrushing techniques,” “motivational interviewing strategies,” and “children.” Boolean operators were strategically utilised to further refine the search results. At the same time, filters were applied to limit the findings to studies published in English, focusing on human populations aged 0-18 years and published between 2000 and 2025.

The methodology's transparency and reproducibility were maintained by adhering to the PRISMA-ScR guidelines (Tricco et al., 2018). A detailed search history, including the specific databases consulted, the keywords used, and the resulting findings, is meticulously documented in Appendix A.

Furthermore, to broaden the scope of the search, grey literature and expert sources were methodically explored through platforms such as Google Scholar, NHS Evidence, and publications from the World Health Organisation (WHO). This effort aimed to uncover relevant research that, although potentially unpublished or not indexed in traditional academic databases, could provide valuable insights into dental nurses' contributions to oral health initiatives for children.

3.7 Study Selection Process

All identified citations were imported into EndNote 21 for de-duplication, followed by data screening using the JBI Data Screening template. Two screening stages were conducted: first, titles and abstracts were reviewed against the inclusion criteria; second, the full texts of potentially eligible studies were assessed in detail. Of the 186 initial records, 24 duplicates were removed. The remaining 162 articles underwent title and abstract screening, with 14 selected for full-text review. Ten studies ultimately met the inclusion criteria. Reasons for exclusion at the full-text stage included a lack of dental nurse involvement, adult-only populations, the absence of caries-related outcomes, or inappropriate study settings. The selection process is summarised in the PRISMA-ScR flow diagram (Figure 4) presented in Chapter 4.

3.8 Data Charting and Extraction

A structured data charting form was created in Microsoft Excel using the JBI Template to extract key information from each included study. Variables included the study title, authorship, publication year, country, design, population, setting, type of intervention, and primary outcomes. The form was pilot tested in two studies and refined to accommodate all relevant data. The process was iterative and aligned with JBI guidance to ensure flexibility in charting emerging themes. A summary of the studies included is presented in Table 1.

3.9 Data Synthesis and Reporting

Data were synthesised using a narrative, thematic synthesis approach, reflecting the scoping nature of the review. Studies were grouped according to intervention type, study setting, and reported outcome. Quantitative data, such as caries reductions, dmft scores, and attendance improvements, were summarised descriptively, while qualitative themes (e.g., barriers, training needs) were presented in context. The synthesis focused on mapping the extent and nature of evidence, rather than assessing quality or effect size, in line with JBI guidance. No meta-analysis was conducted, consistent with the scoping methodology (Levac et al., 2010).

3.10 Critical appraisal of the included articles:

Although critical appraisal is not a formal requirement for scoping reviews, it was conducted in this review to better assess the methodological quality and reliability of the included studies, thereby aiding interpretation of the evidence. This review was intentionally undertaken with an emphasis on interpretive depth, transparency, and readers' understanding of the methodological robustness of the available evidence. Consequently, a two-stage critical appraisal was conducted: the first stage involved an independent review of each article, followed by a second stage that incorporated the relevant items from the JBI checklist to assess the consistency of their application. Each appraisal criterion was marked as "Yes," "No," or "Unclear," with accompanying notes that highlighted the strengths and weaknesses identified.

To ensure reliability and consistency in the appraisal process, the initial appraisals were reviewed and verified for accuracy. When issues arose, the pertinent sections of the full articles were double-checked for accuracy. The same JBI criteria were systematically applied to all studies, thereby minimising subjectivity and enhancing the validity of the quality appraisals.

3.11 Ethical Considerations

As secondary research, this scoping review did not involve human subjects and was exempt from ethics approval. All data were sourced from publicly available documents, with proper reference and adherence to academic integrity principles.

3.12 Summary

This chapter provides a comprehensive overview of the design, execution, and reasoning behind the scoping review. It delves into the search strategy, outlines the inclusion criteria, details the study selection process, and describes the methods used for data synthesis. The methodology was meticulously guided by the renowned JBI and PRISMA-ScR frameworks, ensuring a level of rigour and transparency that underpins the integrity of the review. In the following chapter, we will present the findings, carefully organised to align with the review's objectives, and highlight the key themes that emerged from the analysed studies.

CHAPTER 4: RESULTS

4.1. Introduction:

This chapter clearly presents the results of the scoping review. The first part explains the search technique, including how studies were identified, screened, and selected. The PRISMA flowchart supports this. The chapter describes the features of the studies included and those excluded.

The following section provides a comprehensive summary of the evidence for each objective, highlighting the key findings from each study and identifying gaps in the evidence. The chapter concludes with a critical appraisal of the methodological quality of the studies included and an overall assessment of the evidence.

4.2 Study Search and Screening:

4.2.1 SUMMARY OF THE SEARCH PROCESS:

A systematic search was conducted across four major electronic databases: PubMed, Embase, Scopus, and Web of Science. The initial search yielded 186 entries, comprising 136 from PubMed, 36 from Embase, 7 from Web of Science, and 5 from Scopus. Additionally, a thorough grey literature search across institutional repositories, the reference lists of relevant studies, and the websites of professional dental organisations did not yield any further entries.

All retrieved records were imported into EndNote 21, where 24 duplicates were removed. A total of 162 titles and abstracts were screened against the inclusion and exclusion criteria as described in the study protocol, after de-duplication. This resulted in 14 full-text articles, which were assessed for eligibility. After detailed full-text screening, ten studies were eligible for inclusion in the scoping review.

The PRISMA 2020 flow diagram (Figure 4) shows the step-by-step process for identifying, screening, evaluating eligibility, and including participants in the study. The figure illustrates the number of records found at each stage of the search process and explains why some were excluded from the full-text screening.

Figure 4: The entire search and selection process in the PRISMA flowchart

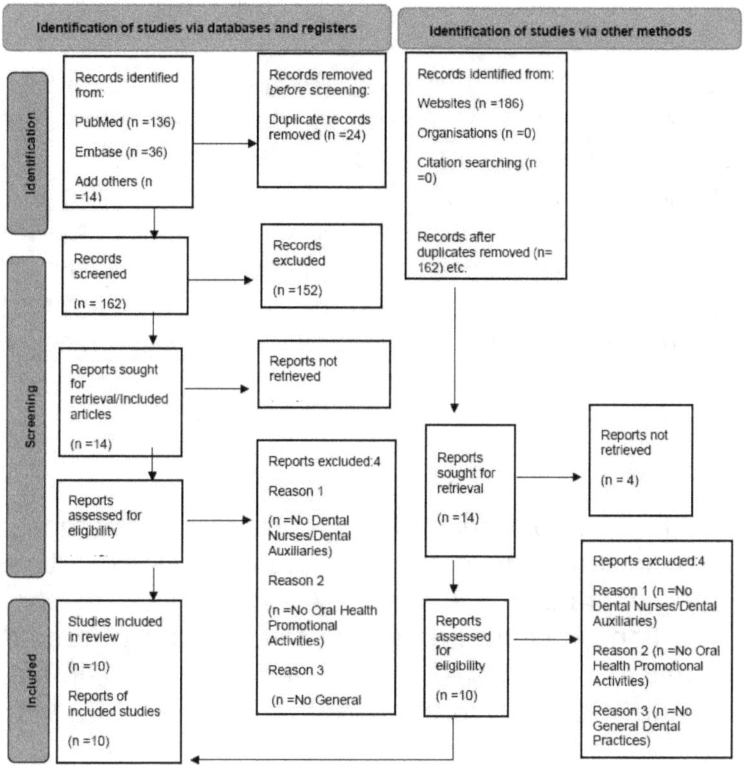

4.2.2 Study Retrieval, Selection, and Exclusion:

During the first phase of the review process, 162 titles and abstracts were screened, and 148 articles were excluded. The primary reasons for exclusion included a lack of focus on dental nurses, insufficient emphasis on preventive interventions, a focus on adult populations, a lack of outcomes related to caries prevention among children, or being classified as editorials rather than original research studies.

Following this initial screen, 14 full-text articles were retrieved and scrutinised in detail with the pre-determined inclusion and exclusion criteria. Ten studies fulfilled all eligibility criteria and were included in the final scoping review. The remaining four full-text articles were excluded for reasons such as the absence of dental nurse-delivered interventions, failure to report caries prevention outcomes of interest, or being editorials.

For the sake of transparency in the selection process, specific reasons for the exclusion of full-text articles were recorded in a study log. A summary of the whole selection process, presenting the number of records identified, screened, excluded, and ultimately included, is given in the modified PRISMA 2020 flow diagram (Figure 1).

The research shows that the majority of studies were conducted in the United Kingdom, with additional studies conducted in the United States, South Africa, and Germany (Figure 5).

The studies were published between 2012 and 2025, reflecting both historical and modern developments in preventive care by dental nurses. The interventions covered in the research included fluoride varnish, oral health education, motivational interviewing, supervised toothbrushing programs, and follow-up outreach activities with families.

4.3 Characteristics of Included Studies:

The ten included studies reflect a range of methodologies (RCT, cross-sectional, before–and–after), geographical settings (UK, Scotland, USA, etc.), and dental nurse-led interventions (fluoride varnish, supervised brushing, motivational interviewing). Most studies were conducted in the UK, reflecting the prominence of dental nurses in the NHS. Study designs included a randomised controlled trial (Pine et al., 2020), a before–and–after study (Howard et al., 2017), a cross-sectional survey (Gnich et al., 2014), and descriptive evaluations (Hatim & Kendall, 2012; O'Keefe, 2015). Several program evaluations (Kidd et al., 2020; Ross et al., 2023) and reviews (Peerbhay et al., 2025; Gallagher et al., 2024) were also included. Interventions examined across these studies ranged from motivational interviewing and fluoride varnish application to supervised brushing and dietary counselling. Outcomes varied, including clinical measures (e.g., dmft scores), behavioural outcomes (e.g., brushing frequency), and service-related metrics (e.g., improved attendance). See Table 3 for complete details.

Figure 5: Countries where included studies were conducted, showing the global distribution of evidence on dental nurse-led caries prevention.

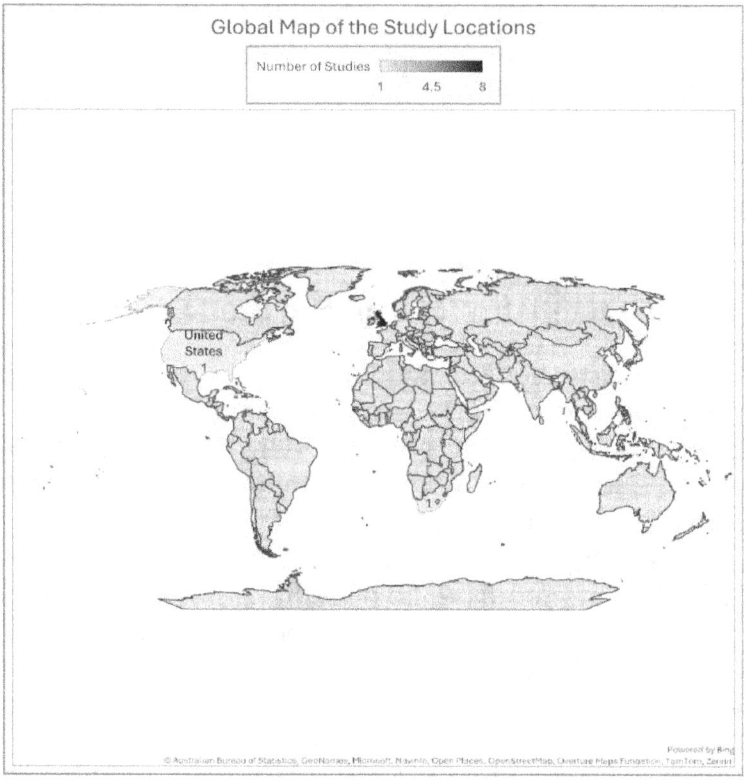

The primary outcomes measured included changes in dental caries (caries increment), as reflected in dmft scores. Intermediate outcomes were also measured, including improvements in dental attendance and increased confidence among dental nurses. Studies also collected qualitative data from dental nurses, parents, and children on the acceptability, feasibility, and perceived barriers to preventive interventions.

Objective 1: Dental Nurses' Oral Health Promotion Activities in General Dental Practices Worldwide:

Among the studies included, dental nurses delivered a range of oral health promotion and preventive interventions in general dental practice. Routine activities comprised the delivery of fluoride varnish application (Hatim & Kendall, 2012; Pine et al., 2020; Howard et al., 2017; Ross et al., 2023; Kidd et al., 2020), oral health education sessions (O'Keefe, 2015; Conway & Burns, 2014), and, in some instances, motivational interviewing (Pine et al., 2020).

One study reported the use of outreach programs, including follow-up telephone communication, to improve appointment compliance and reinforce oral health education (Gehsan & Mijic, 2019). However, none of these studies reported actual examples of dental nurses conducting caries risk assessments independently or applying fissure sealants in general dental practice. None of the studies reviewed considered the use of digital tools or apps in the delivery of oral health education by dental nurses. Figure 6 illustrates that the majority of activities focused on oral health education.

Figure 6: Types of nurse-led interventions reported across included studies showing the frequency of each preventive approach delivered by dental nurses in general dental practice.

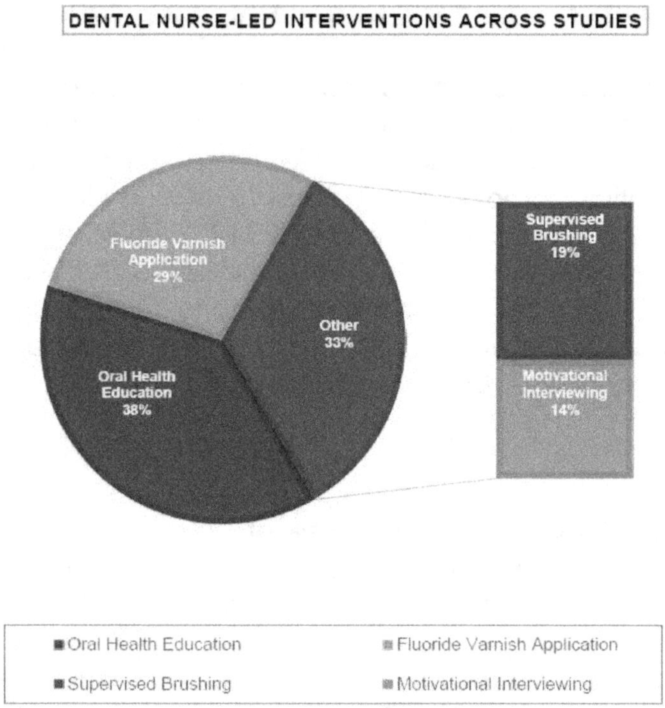

Objective 2: Groups of Children Targeted by Dental Nurses

Most of the research has targeted children known to be at high risk for dental caries, including those who live in areas of high socioeconomic disadvantage (Howard et al., 2017; Ross et al., 2023; Kidd et al., 2020) and those who required dental treatment under general anaesthesia because of widespread decay (Pine et al., 2020). Two studies have involved larger samples of children attending general dental practices for regular check-ups (Hatim & Kendall, 2012; O'Keefe, 2015); however, detailed demographic information, such as family income, ethnicity, or parental education, was not typically provided. Furthermore, none of the studies aimed explicitly for children with disabilities or special healthcare needs, which indicates a significant gap within the existing evidence. The measured outcomes are discussed in the following section.

Objective 3: Outcomes Measured in Studies Featuring Dental Nurses:

The outcomes assessed showed significant variation among the studies examined. Clinical outcomes, such as reductions in mean dmft scores or the development of new caries, were reported in research carried out by Pine et al. (2020), Howard et al. (2017), Ross et al. (2023), and Kidd et al. (2020). There was only one RCT that assessed caries increment (Pine et al, 2020).

Intermediate results included improved appointment attendance rates (Gehsan & Mijic, 2019) and increased confidence levels among dental nurses after training (Hatim & Kendall, 2012). Qualitative results were also reported, including dental nurses' assessments of training quality, barriers in the delivery of preventive care, and families' responses to education visits (O'Keefe, 2015; Conway & Burns, 2014). However, some studies did not have an extensive measurement of parents' or children's behavioural change, while none provided long-term follow-up on the maintenance of oral health behaviour improvements. The evidence showed that outcomes measured were heterogeneous, with few studies assessing long-term behavioural change, thus limiting the knowledge about the long-lasting impacts of interventions. The last aim appraises the effectiveness of these interventions.

Objective 4: Effectiveness of Dental Nurse-Led Interventions:

Among the included studies, the most substantial evidence for effectiveness came from the Randomised Controlled Trial (RCT) by Pine et al. (2020), which evaluated the impact of a nurse-delivered intervention on caries development among high-risk children. The study included 241 children aged 5–7 years attending general dental practices in England. The intervention group received fluoride varnish applications twice yearly, coupled with motivational interviewing (MI) delivered by trained dental nurses, while the control group received standard care. After a 24-month follow-up, the mean dmft score in the intervention group was 1.02 (SD = 0.91), compared to 1.71 (SD = 1.23) in the control group (**29% relative reduction in new caries incidence** and a **51% lower odds of recurrence** compared with a control conversation), indicating a significant reduction in caries increment ($p < 0.01$). This study demonstrates the effectiveness of targeted, nurse-led preventive care when supported by behavioural change strategies.

In contrast, cross-sectional studies—such as those by Howard et al. (2017), Ross et al. (2023), and Kidd et al. (2020)—assessed the associations between nurse-led interventions and oral health outcomes. These studies reported positive trends in caries reduction and attendance among children attending practices with ongoing involvement from a dental nurse. However, none of these studies included control groups or follow-up data, limiting the ability to attribute observed outcomes directly to the intervention.

One before-and-after study by Howard et al. (2017) evaluated the effect of dental nurse-delivered fluoride varnish and toothbrushing advice in a sample of 356 children aged 3–6 years. The study reported a 12% reduction in untreated caries rates after 12 months. However, without a comparison group, it is challenging to exclude external influences such as community campaigns or other concurrent practice-based efforts.

Finally, descriptive studies, such as those by Hatim & Kendall (2012), O'Keefe (2015), and Conway & Burns (2014), have described dental nurse-led interventions (e.g., parent education sessions, supervised brushing, and school visits). Still, they did not quantify effectiveness or provide baseline/follow-up data. Therefore, their contributions to caries prevention, while promising in narrative, cannot be confirmed without stronger study designs. These findings underscore the need for more rigorous evaluations of nurse-led interventions, with a focus on well-defined outcomes, control groups, and extended follow-up periods. Figure 7 shows the distribution of studies based on review objectives, emphasising oral health promotion, fluoride varnish application, and dietary advice.

Figure 7: Distribution of Studies According to Review Objectives

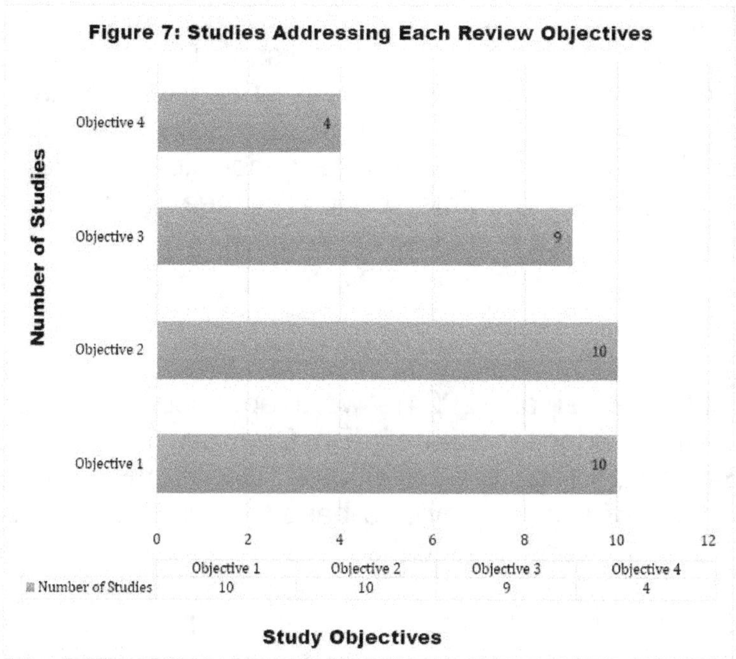

4.4 Quality Evaluation and Critical Appraisal of the Studies Included:

Howard et al. (2017), Ross et al. (2023), and Kidd et al. (2020) were assessed using the JBI Checklist for Analytical Cross-Sectional Studies, which includes clearly defined inclusion criteria, the validity and reliability of exposure and outcome measures, the identification of confounders, and the use of appropriate statistical analysis.

Hatim & Kendall (2012), O'Keefe (2015), Conway & Burns (2014), and Gehsan & Mijic (2019) were appraised using the JBI Checklist for Case Series or Descriptive Studies. The checklist explicitly looks for clearly defined cases, accurate reporting of participant demographics, consecutive inclusion, detailed descriptions of interventions, measurement of outcomes, and complete follow-up.

Two included reviews—Peerbhay et al. (2025) and Gallagher et al. (2024)—were appraised using the Joanna Briggs Institute (JBI) Checklist for Scoping Reviews. This tool evaluates the methodological quality of scoping reviews based on criteria such as the clarity and justification of inclusion criteria, the comprehensiveness of the search strategy, the transparency of data extraction methods, and the appropriateness of the synthesis and presentation of findings. While both reviews explored a range of oral health promotion interventions involving dental nurses, they also noted considerable heterogeneity among the included studies and a lack of standardised outcome measures. These limitations reduce the ability to draw firm conclusions about the effectiveness of nurse-led interventions and reinforce the need for more rigorously designed primary research in this area.

A two-stage critical appraisal was conducted: the first was an independent screening of each article, followed by a second review that included the respective JBI checklist items to determine consistency of application. Each appraisal criterion was marked as "Yes," "No," or "Unclear," with notes documenting the strengths and weaknesses identified.

To ensure reliability and consistency in the appraisal process, the first few appraisals were reviewed and verified for accuracy. Wherever issues arose, the relevant sections of the full articles were verified twice. The same JBI criteria were systematically applied to all studies; therefore, subjectivity was minimised, and the validity of the quality appraisals was enhanced. Table 5 provides a summary of the methodological quality of all included studies, based on the appropriate JBI critical appraisal tools.

Table 5: Table of Evidence Quality Appraisal Summary

Study	Design	Quality Appraisal Summary
Pine et al. (2020)	RCT	High, randomisation and valid outcomes; blinding not reported
Howard et al. (2017)	Cross-Sectional	Moderate; large sample, valid measures; confounders not adjusted
Ross et al. (2023)	Cross-Sectional	Moderate; robust outcomes; limited subgroup reporting
Kidd et al. (2020)	Cross-Sectional	Moderate; appropriate analysis; partial confounder consideration
Hatim & Kendall (2012)	Case Series	Low; descriptive only, lacked objective outcomes and standardised delivery.
O'Keefe (2015)	Case Series	Low: small sample, subjective outcomes, unclear sample selection
Conway & Burns (2014)	Case Series	Low; no clinical outcomes, limited intervention details
Gehsan & Mijic (2019)	Case Series	Low; focus on attendance improvements, no direct clinical measures

Peerbhay et al. (2025)	Scoping Rev.	Moderate; rigorous methods, with limited heterogeneity, allowing for conclusions specific to dental nurses.
Gallagher et al. (2024	Rapid Rev.	Moderate; clear methods, lacked direct evaluation of nurse-led interventions.

Pine et al. (2020) fulfilled almost all JBI RCT criteria, including the generation of a random sequence (adequate), comparability of the intervention and control groups at baseline, a valid and reliable outcome measurement (incidence of new caries), and complete follow-up. It did not, however, report whether the outcome assessors were blinded, a potential source of detection bias.

The three cross-sectional studies (Howard et al. (2017), Ross et al. (2023), Kidd et al. (2020) were characterised by large sample sizes and the use of validated outcome measures (namely, dmft/d3mft scores) that worked to increase internal consistency and reliability. These studies, however, neglected to control for or include notable confounding variables known to have independent effects on caries outcomes, such as dietary habits, socioeconomic status, and oral hygiene practices outside the clinical setting. While the statistical methods used were generally applicable, the lack of reporting on demographic variables limited the ability to determine subgroup effects.

The four descriptive studies (Hatim & Kendall, 2012; O'Keefe, 2015; Conway & Burns, 2014; Gehsan & Mijic, 2019) provided valuable qualitative insights into perceptions, levels of confidence, and everyday experiences of nurses engaged in interventions such as fluoride varnish application and oral health promotion. However, the studies were marked by the lack of control groups, difficulties related to measuring and quantifying objective clinical outcomes (e.g., caries incidence), and either small or unclear sample sizes; there was no claim that all eligible patients had been approached consecutively for inclusion. The lack of sufficient demographic data also limited the ability to determine representativeness or generalizability.

The scoping and rapid reviews employed extensive search strategies, were based on explicit inclusion criteria, and were guided by systematic selection processes, thereby meeting the vast majority of the JBI guidelines for systematic reviews. The reviews, however, were flawed by considerable heterogeneity among included studies in their designs, interventions, and outcomes, which restricted the scope of the reviews for conducting a quantitative synthesis to any significant degree or for providing coherent and firm conclusions about the effectiveness of interventions carried out independently by dental nurses.

4.5 Limitations:

The studies reviewed demonstrated some methodological weaknesses. The use of small or poorly described sample sizes in much descriptive work thus threatens the credibility and generalizability of the results. The absence of control or comparison groups in non-randomised studies meant that observed effects could not be confidently attributed to interventions delivered by dental nurses. In addition, interventions were often implemented without a standardised protocol, raising concerns about the fidelity and consistency of the intervention as delivered to participants. In most cases, short or absent follow-up periods precluded assessment of the longevity of observed effects. In cross-sectional studies, failure to define or control for putative confounding factors—e.g., dietary habits, oral hygiene behaviours outside the clinical environment, and socioeconomic status—also undermined internal validity. The absence of demographic information, such as socioeconomic and ethnic data, limited the potential to assess the effectiveness of interventions in the broader population or to address recognised disparities in health outcomes. Notably, no research has expressly examined interventions provided by dental nurses to disabled children or those with special healthcare needs, a significant omission in the existing evidence base. Taken together, these shortcomings reduce the confidence with which conclusions may be reached and highlight the pressing need for more rigorous and extensive research in this field.

To visually synthesise the distribution of evidence across the four scoping review objectives and the preventive roles performed by dental nurses, a combined bar chart was created (Figure 8). This figure shows that the majority of studies focused on describing dental nurse roles and their preventive activities, with considerably fewer studies focusing on effectiveness, barriers to implementation, or training-related aspects. The figure also illustrates the varied frequency of different interventions—such as fluoride varnish application, oral health education, supervised toothbrushing, and motivational interviewing—within each objective. It highlights that fluoride varnish and OHE were the most frequently studied, whereas dietary counselling and outreach interventions were underrepresented across all objectives.

This visual synthesis confirms that while specific interventions are well established in practice, others have not received equal attention in research, particularly regarding effectiveness or long-term implementation. This imbalance highlights the need for a comprehensive evaluation of dental nurse-led activities across the full spectrum to support the evidence-informed expansion of their preventive roles.

In conclusion, these findings emphasise the importance of conducting future research with rigorous, controlled designs that utilise standardised intervention protocols. It's essential to have longer follow-up periods, thorough evaluation of both clinical and behavioural outcomes, and meticulous documentation of demographic information. This approach will strengthen the evidence supporting the role of dental nurses in delivering caries-prevention strategies for children.

Figure 8. Combined Bar Chart Showing Distribution of Dental Nurse-Led Preventive Interventions across the four review objectives.

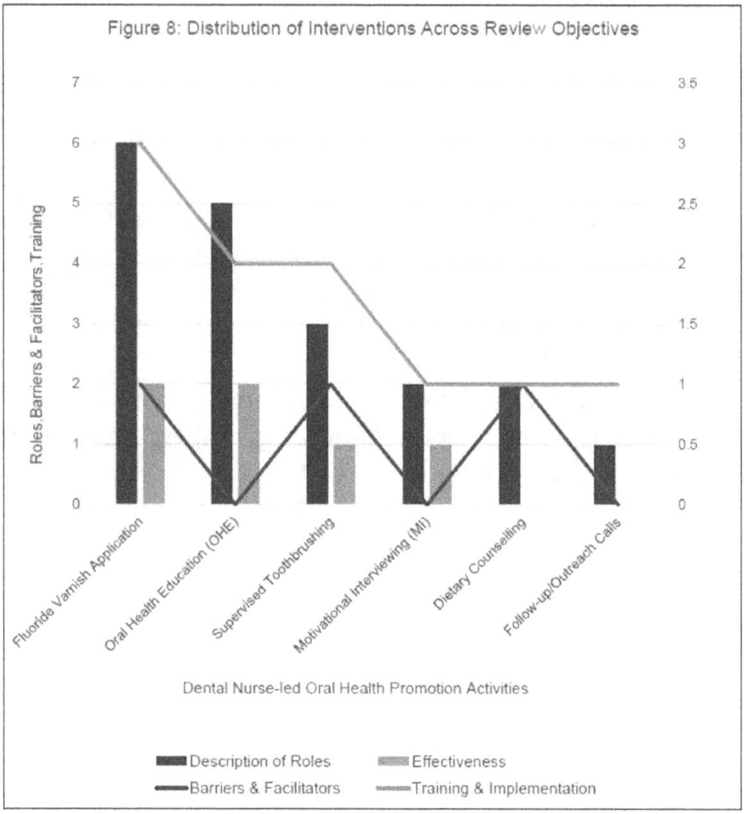

4.6. Evaluation of the Evidence:

The randomised controlled trial conducted by Pine et al. (2020) stands out as the most compelling source of evidence regarding the effectiveness of dental nurse-led interventions. In contrast, the descriptive and cross-sectional studies have offered valuable insights into the various components and delivery methods of these interventions. Notably, Pine et al. discovered that children who received fluoride varnish treatments accompanied by nurse-led motivational interviewing exhibited a statistically significant decrease in the incidence of new cavities. This finding suggests that interventions led by dental nurses can effectively prevent cavities in children. However, it is crucial to point out that the overall body of evidence is somewhat limited, as the majority of existing studies have primarily focused on oral health education initiatives within the UK.

The quality of the methodologies employed across these studies varied, with many falling into the moderate to low-quality category. A significant number of descriptive studies relied heavily on qualitative feedback or self-reported outcomes, which often lack the precision and reliability provided by objective measures of treatment effectiveness. Moreover, many studies did not utilise standardised intervention protocols or include control groups, and they frequently failed to provide clear accounts of participants' characteristics. This lack of rigour makes it challenging to determine whether the reported positive outcomes were entirely attributable to the nurse-led interventions. Additionally, substantial differences in study designs, intervention types, outcomes assessed, and populations studied create challenges for drawing direct comparisons and reaching consistent conclusions across the existing literature.

It is also essential to note that none of the studies specifically focused on dental nurse-led care for children with disabilities or those with special healthcare needs. Furthermore, many studies lacked detailed demographic data, including information about participants' racial backgrounds and socioeconomic status. This omission diminishes our ability to evaluate the equity and generalizability of the interventions' effectiveness.

The evidence suggests that dental nurses can play a crucial role in preventing cavities among children by providing comprehensive preventive care. However, the significant proportion of research characterised by moderate to low quality highlights the urgent need for more rigorously designed studies. Future research should prioritise robust methodologies, such as randomised controlled trials with larger, more diverse samples, standardised intervention protocols, thorough outcome assessments, and extended follow-up periods. These enhancements will be crucial in determining the long-term effectiveness of dental nurse-led interventions in general dental practices and a wider array of healthcare settings. The next chapter, titled "Discussion," will further explore these findings, compare them with existing knowledge, and investigate their implications for health policy, clinical practice, and directions for future research.

4.7 Summary

This scoping review identified 10 relevant studies highlighting the growing role of dental nurses in providing preventive oral health care. While the evidence is promising, it is limited by study quality, inconsistent reporting, and a narrow focus on specific populations. These findings are discussed in greater detail in Chapter 5, which explores the implications for practice, policy, and research.

CHAPTER 5: DISCUSSION

5.1 Overview of Main Findings

This scoping review aimed to comprehensively evaluate the global evidence on the preventive roles of dental nurses in general dental practices, particularly those focusing on children. The review included 10 studies that highlighted the proactive involvement of dental nurses in initiatives to prevent dental caries. These initiatives encompassed a range of interventions, including the application of fluoride varnish, oral health education, supervised toothbrushing, dietary counselling to promote healthier eating habits, and motivational interviewing to encourage positive behavioural changes in children.

Despite the promising roles of dental nurses illustrated in these studies, the review revealed considerable variability in both the scope and methodological rigour of the evidence presented. Most studies were either descriptive or observational, with only a single well-designed randomised controlled trial available to rigorously assess clinical outcomes. Additionally, the studies varied significantly in terms of the specific populations they targeted, ranging from different age groups to diverse socioeconomic backgrounds, and the outcomes they measured. There was also a notable lack of long-term follow-up data, limiting the ability to draw generalizable conclusions about the effectiveness of these interventions across settings.

5.2 Interpretation in the Context of Existing Literature

The findings align with previous literature indicating that dental nurses, particularly those trained in extended duties, are well-positioned to support prevention in primary care (GDC, 2023; Anderson et al., 2020). The predominance of fluoride varnish and oral health education reflects the activities most commonly delegated to dental nurses under current UK policy, as supported by Delivering Better Oral Health (OHID, 2021). However, more advanced techniques—such as motivational interviewing or digital health tools—remain under-researched, despite their potential in behaviour change and caries prevention.

The reviewed studies rarely disaggregated dental nurse-led outcomes from those of broader team-based interventions. In multi-component programmes like Childsmile (Kidd et al., 2020), the effectiveness of the dental nurse role is often embedded in systemic change, making it difficult to isolate individual contributions. This lack of role-specific outcome measurement limits policy-relevant conclusions and highlights a fundamental research gap.

Furthermore, consistent with Watt and Sheiham's (2012) argument for addressing the social determinants of oral health, few studies included children from ethnically diverse or socioeconomically deprived groups. None explicitly focused on children with special healthcare needs, an omission also observed in recent policy critiques (OHID, 2021).

5.3. Strength and Distribution of Evidence

While some high-quality studies exist, notably the randomised controlled trial by Pine et al. (2020), which assessed a dental nurse-led behavioural intervention (DR-BNI) involving 241 children and demonstrated a reduction in caries recurrence, many studies in this area are descriptive or observational. Systematic reviews by Peerbhay et al. (2025) and Gallagher et al. (2024) have highlighted the potential roles of dental nurses but concluded that many of the included studies were heterogeneous and lacked a rigorous evaluation of intervention effectiveness. This review also echoed those findings: only a few studies utilised standardised protocols or included control groups, and many lacked longitudinal follow-up.

5.4 Methodological Limitations of the Included Studies

A critical examination of the study designs revealed several limitations in the current evidence base. Descriptive articles, such as those by Hatim & Kendall (2012) and O'Keefe (2015), outline dental nurse-led interventions. Still, they failed to measure their impact on clinical outcomes or behaviours, making it challenging to conclude effectiveness. Cross-sectional evaluations, such as those by Ross et al. (2023) and Kidd et al. (2020), reported associations between national programmes (e.g., Childsmile) and caries reduction, but did not isolate the contribution of dental nurses or use control groups. Furthermore, before-and-after studies, such as those by Howard et al. (2017), lacked follow-up durations sufficient to establish sustained change and often did not report detailed data (e.g., dmft scores with standard deviations or statistical significance testing).

As a result, the overall quality of evidence was judged to be moderate to low, with a heavy reliance on descriptive and non-comparative designs. Only one study (Pine et al., 2020) employed a randomised design with defined outcomes and follow-up periods, providing more substantial evidence for the role of dental nurses. The lack of robust quantitative data across most studies limits the strength of conclusions that can be drawn from the collective findings.

5.5 Public Health and Policy Implications

Despite methodological limitations, the findings have clear implications for public health planning and workforce development. Dental nurses represent a cost-effective and scalable asset in delivering evidence-based oral health promotion. By expanding their scope through certified training in interventions such as OHE and fluoride varnish application, general dental practices can shift toward prevention-led care pathways.

Policies that support the upskilling and recognition of dental nurses—particularly through Continuing Professional Development (CPD), financial incentives, and supervision protocols—could enhance service delivery. NHS frameworks, such as Flexible Commissioning and the recent Dental Recovery Plan (NHS England, 2023), already endorse the use of skill mix, but implementation remains inconsistent. Strengthening this alignment between policy and practice is essential to relieve pressure on dentists and widen access to care.

However, the lack of economic evaluations within the reviewed literature limits the ability to advocate for broader policy reform. Future studies must integrate cost-effectiveness metrics and assess scalability, particularly in underserved or high-need populations.

5.6 Research Gaps and Future Recommendations

This review has brought to light several critical areas of research that warrant further empirical investigation and exploration:

First, while the addition of high-quality randomised controlled trials (RCTs) could significantly bolster the evidence base for specific preventive interventions delivered by dental nurses, the current findings suggest that the challenge may extend beyond a lack of evidence. A primary focus for both research and policy should be directed toward enhancing training programs, fostering workforce development, and expanding the scope of practice for dental nurses, enabling them to function at their full potential. Such measures could empower dental nurses to play a more proactive role in patient care and preventive strategies.

In the UK context, several systemic barriers hinder dental nurses' progress in undertaking expanded roles and responsibilities. These barriers include stringent NHS contracts, which often dictate the parameters of care delivery; limited commissioning of services led by dental nurses, with a focus on preventive measures; and the frequent underutilization of a skilled mix within dental practices. These challenges can prevent dental nurses from undertaking tasks that research has shown to be effective in improving patient outcomes. Therefore, future research should examine implementation strategies, advocate for policy reforms, and assess the cost-effectiveness of expanding dental nurses' roles within the NHS. Such investigations could be equally as important as conducting additional RCTs.

Second, future research endeavours should aim to disentangle the specific contributions of dental nurses from those of other healthcare team members, particularly in multidisciplinary initiatives such as Childsmile. Understanding the unique impacts of dental nurses will be essential in measuring their effectiveness in improving oral health outcomes among different populations.

Third, there is a pressing need for more qualitative and mixed-methods research to examine the barriers and facilitators influencing nurse-led interventions. By capturing patient perspectives and assessing their acceptability, researchers can better inform strategies to encourage their wider implementation.

Fourth, a significant gap identified in this review is the absence of formal economic analyses in the studies reviewed. Conducting cost-effectiveness evaluations is crucial for guiding policy decisions and workforce planning, ultimately ensuring that resources are allocated efficiently and that interventions yield sustainable benefits.

Ultimately, future research should consider equity outcomes, specifically examining whether dental nurse-led preventive initiatives reduce disparities in oral health among children. This includes focusing on those from ethnically diverse backgrounds, economically disadvantaged families, and those with special educational needs and disabilities (SEND). By addressing these equity concerns, we can work toward ensuring that all children have access to effective oral health prevention strategies.

5.7 Summary

The findings of this scoping review demonstrate that dental nurses are increasingly involved in delivering preventive oral health interventions for children in general dental practices. However, the evidence supporting these roles is mixed, with strong findings from a limited number of studies (e.g., Pine et al., 2020) but generally low methodological quality across the literature. While fluoride varnish and OHE interventions are commonly reported, other strategies remain underexplored. The current evidence base, although promising, is insufficiently rigorous to inform national-scale service redesigns. To realise the full preventive potential of dental nurses, further investment in research, training, and implementation support is urgently required.

CHAPTER 6: CONCLUSION AND RECOMMENDATIONS

6.1 Conclusion

This scoping review examined global evidence on the role of dental nurses in delivering oral health promotion (OHP) interventions to prevent dental caries in children in general dental practices. Ten studies met the inclusion criteria, most of which originated from high-income countries and described preventive interventions, including fluoride varnish application, oral health education, supervised toothbrushing, and motivational interviewing. These findings suggest that dental nurses, particularly those trained in extended duties, are making a meaningful contribution to the prevention of early childhood caries, especially within NHS general dental practice settings.

However, the existing literature is limited by methodological variability, small sample sizes, inconsistent reporting of outcomes, and a lack of studies from low- and middle-income countries. Only one included study used a randomised controlled trial design to evaluate a dental nurse-led intervention. Furthermore, many studies have failed to disaggregate the role of dental nurses from that of other dental team members, making it difficult to determine their unique contribution. These limitations reflect the broader challenges in assessing the effectiveness of skill-mix in dentistry and highlight a need for more targeted, high-quality research. Despite these gaps, this review supports the growing consensus that dental nurses are well-placed to support caries prevention through structured, evidence-based health promotion interventions. National guidelines and workforce strategies increasingly endorse their involvement, but practice remains inconsistent across regions and settings. These findings underscore the importance of integrating dental nurses more effectively into primary oral health care teams and highlight the need for enhanced documentation, training, and recognition of their roles across dental services.

6.2 Recommendations

To strengthen the integration and impact of dental nurses in caries prevention, several recommendations are proposed for practice, policy, education, and research.

In clinical practice, dental nurses should be routinely involved in delivering oral health promotion services, such as fluoride varnish application, oral hygiene instruction, and dietary counselling. Their participation should be formally incorporated into standard recall appointments, where they can reinforce preventive messages through behaviour change strategies tailored to children and their families.

At the policy level, there is a clear need for national dental commissioning frameworks to recognise and incentivise dental nurses' preventive roles formally. This includes updating contracts to allow for extended duties, introducing measurable quality outcomes related to prevention, and ensuring financial support for workforce development. In particular, health authorities should prioritise dental nurse-led initiatives in areas with high rates of untreated caries or limited access to paediatric dental services.

From an educational standpoint, the dental nursing training curriculum should be updated to include modules on evidence-based prevention, health communication, and motivational interviewing techniques. In addition, Continuing Professional Development (CPD) programmes should support practising dental nurses in expanding their skill set to deliver practical, child-centred health promotion. Ensuring consistency in training across the NHS and private sectors will help standardise care delivery and increase confidence in the preventive role of dental nurses.

Further research is urgently needed to build a more robust evidence base. Future studies should employ rigorous designs, such as randomised controlled trials and longitudinal cohort studies, to evaluate both clinical and behavioural outcomes associated with dental nurse-led interventions. Research should also explore the cost-effectiveness and scalability of these models to inform service planning. Importantly, more studies should focus on underserved or high-risk populations, including children with special educational needs, those from low-income families, and ethnically diverse communities. Qualitative and mixed-methods research can provide valuable insight into the acceptability, barriers, and facilitators of these interventions from the perspectives of patients, families, and dental professionals.

6.3 Final Reflection

This review has demonstrated that dental nurses play a valuable but often underutilised role in promoting oral health and preventing dental caries among children. Their involvement in delivering preventive interventions within general dental practices represents an opportunity to alleviate workforce pressures, improve access to care, and reduce oral health inequalities. However, limitations in current evidence—particularly the scarcity of high-quality, nurse-specific data—limit our ability to understand their impact fully. For dental nurses to achieve their full potential in supporting children's oral health, investment is needed in training, role development, and targeted research. With the proper support, dental nurses can play a central role in the future of prevention-focused, team-based dental care.

Implications for Practice, Policy, and Future Research

This book highlights the critical yet underutilised role of dental nurses in delivering oral health promotion activities to prevent dental caries in children within general dental practices. The findings support integrating dental nurses into prevention-focused models of care, particularly through structured training, precise role definitions, and supportive practice environments.

From a practice perspective, greater utilisation of dental nurses may improve efficiency, enhance patient engagement, and support continuity of preventive care for children and families. From a policy perspective, aligning commissioning frameworks, workforce planning, and training opportunities with prevention-led care models may strengthen the delivery of equitable oral health services.

Future research should prioritise robust study designs, including randomised controlled trials and longitudinal evaluations, to assess the long-term effectiveness and cost-effectiveness of dental nurse-led interventions. Greater attention should also be given to underserved populations, including children with special healthcare needs and those from socioeconomically disadvantaged backgrounds.

6.4 Conflicts of Interest:

No conflicts of interest were identified. Sources were objectively evaluated, and inclusion decisions were in accordance with the JBI criteria for scoping reviews. Potential bias from prior experience was mitigated through a transparent search and appraisal process.

6.5 Funding:

No external funding was received for this research. The absence of funding reduced the risk of funding-related bias.

References and Bibliography:

Anderson, R., Treasure, E. T. and White, D., 2020. Promoting oral health in primary dental care. Community Dental Health, 37(4), pp. 261–268.

Arksey, H. and O'Malley, L., 2005. Scoping studies: Towards a methodological framework. International Journal of Social Research Methodology, 8(1), pp. 19–32.

Barker, T. H., Habibi, N., Aromataris, E., Stone, J. C., Leonardi-Bee, J., Sears, K., et al., 2024. The revised JBI critical appraisal tool for the assessment of risk of bias in quasi-experimental studies. JBI Evidence Synthesis, 22(3), pp. 378–388.

Cooper, A., O'Malley, L., Elison, S. N. and Worthington, H. V. (2013) 'Primary school-based behavioural interventions for preventing caries'. Cochrane Database of Systematic Reviews, (5).

Eaton, K., Yusuf, H. and Vassallo, P., 2023. The WHO Global Oral Health Action Plan 2023-2030. Community Dental Health, 40(2), pp.68-69.

GBD, 2019. Global Burden of Disease Study 2019: Results. [online] Available at: https://vizhub.healthdata.org/gbd-results/ [Accessed 10 July 2025].

Gehshan, S. and Mijic, M., 2011. Getting Help for Children: The Need to Expand the Dental Workforce. Journal of the California Dental Association, 39(7), pp. 481-490.

GDC (2024). Scope of Practice. [online] General Dental Council. Available at: https://www.gdc-uk.org/standards-guidance/standards-and-guidance/scope-of-practice.

Gnich, W., Deas, L., Mackenzie, S., Burns, J. and Conway, D. I., 2014. Extending dental nurses' duties: a national survey investigating skill-mix in Scotland's child oral health improvement programme (Childsmile). BMC Oral Health, 14(1), p. 137.

Harris, R., Nicoll, A. D., Adair, P. M. and Pine, C. M. (2012) 'Risk factors for dental caries in young children: a systematic review of longitudinal studies'. Community Dental Health, 21(1), pp. 71–85.

Hatim, E. and Kendall, N., 2012. Barriers encountered when using a skill-mix approach to deliver caries prevention in dental practices. Primary Dental Care, (2), pp. 53-57.

Joanna Briggs Institute (2020). Critical Appraisal Tools. [online] JBI. Available at: https://jbi.global/critical-appraisal-tools.

Kidd, J. B., McMahon, A. D., Sherriff, A., Gnich, W., Mahmoud, A., Macpherson, L. M. and Conway, D. I., 2020. Evaluation of a national complex oral health improvement programme: a population data linkage cohort study in Scotland. BMJ open, 10(11), p. e038116.

Kouassi, S. M., Salomon-Ibarra, C. C., Hosey, M. T. and Gallagher, J. E., 2024. Effectiveness of preventive intervention programmes aiming to improve oral health in children who have undergone caries-related dental extractions: a rapid review. Community Dental Health, 41(3), pp. 208-214.

Levac, D., Colquhoun, H. and O'Brien, K. K., 2010. Scoping studies: Advancing the methodology. Implementation Science, 5(1), p. 69.

Lockwood, C., Munn, Z. and Porritt, K., 2020. Chapter 2: Systematic reviews of qualitative evidence. In:

Aromataris, E. and Munn, Z., eds. JBI Manual for Evidence Synthesis. Adelaide: JBI.

Marinho, V. C., Worthington, H. V., Walsh, T. and Clarkson, J. E., 2016. Fluoride varnishes are used to prevent dental caries in children and adolescents—Cochrane Database of Systematic Reviews, (7).

Moola S, Munn Z, Tufanaru C, Aromataris E, Sears K, Sfetcu R, Currie M, Lisy K, Qureshi R, Mattis P, Mu P. Systematic reviews of etiology and risk (2020). Aromataris E, Lockwood C, Porritt K, Pilla B, Jordan Z, editors. JBI Manual for Evidence Synthesis. JBI; 2024. Available from: https://synthesismanual.jbi.global. https://doi.org/10.46658/JBIMES-24-06 .

NICE (2015). Oral health promotion: general dental practice NICE guideline. [online] Available at: https://www.nice.org.uk/guidance/ng30/resources/oral-health-promotion-general-dental-practice-pdf-1837385644741.

O'Keefe, E., 2015. Communication skills for extended duties dental nurses: the childsmile perspective. Primary dental journal, 4(1), pp. 64-66.

Department of Health and Social care (2021). Delivering better oral health: an evidence-based toolkit for prevention. [online] GOV.UK. Available at: https://www.gov.uk/government/publications/delivering-better-oral-health-an-evidence-based-toolkit-for-prevention.

Page, M. J., McKenzie, J. E., Bossuyt, P. M., Boutron, I., Hoffmann, T. C., Mulrow, C. D., et al., 2021. The PRISMA 2020 statement: An updated guideline for reporting systematic reviews. BMJ, 372, p. n71.

Peerbhay, F., Mash, R. and Khan, S., 2025. Effectiveness of oral health promotion in children and adolescents through behaviour change interventions: a scoping review. Plos one, 20(1), p. e0316702.

Peters, M. D. J., Marnie, C., Colquhoun, H., Garritty, C., Hempel, S., Horsley, T., et al., 2020. Updated methodological guidance for the conduct of scoping reviews. JBI Evidence Synthesis, 18(10), pp. 2119–2126. https://doi. org/10. 11124/JBIES-20-00167

Peters MDJ, Godfrey C, McInerney P, Munn Z, Tricco AC, Khalil, H. Chapter 11: Scoping Reviews (2020 version). In: Aromataris E, Munn Z (Editors). JBI, 2020. Available JBI Manual for Evidence Synthesis from https://synthesismanual.jbi.global . https://doi.org/10.46658/JBIMES-20-12

Petersen, P.E., Bourgeois, D., Ogawa, H., Estupinan-Day, S. and Ndiaye, C., 2005. The global burden of oral diseases and risks to oral health. Bulletin of the world health organization, 83, pp.661-669.

Public Health England (2023). National Dental Epidemiology Programme (NDEP) for England: oral health survey of 5 year old children 2022. [online] GOV.UK. Available at: https://www.gov.uk/government/statistics/oral-health-survey-of-5-year-old-children-2022/national-dental-epidemiology-programme-ndep-for-england-oral-health-survey-of-5-year-old-children-2022.

Pine, C. M., Adair, P. M., Burnside, G., Brennan, L., Sutton, L., Edwards, R. T., Ezeofor, V., Albadri, S., Curnow, M. M., Deery, C. and Hosey, M. T., 2020. Dental RECUR randomised trial to prevent caries recurrence in children. Journal of Dental Research, 99(2), pp. 168-174.

Public Health England (2018). Oral health survey of 5 year old children 2017. [online] GOV.UK. Available at: https://www.gov.uk/government/statistics/oral-health-survey-of-5-year-old-children-2017.

Ribeiro, A., Silva, M., Martelli, P. and Leles, C. (2014) 'Oral health promotion in primary care: The role of dental auxiliaries in low-income settings'. BMC Oral Health, 14(1), p. 66.

Ross, A. J., Sherriff, A., Kidd, J., Deas, L., Eaves, J., Blokland, A., Wright, B., King, P., McMahon, A. D., Conway, D. I. and Macpherson, L. M., 2023. Evaluating childsmile, Scotland's National Oral Health Improvement Programme for children. Community Dentistry and Oral Epidemiology, 51(1), pp. 133-138.

SDCEP (2011). Oral Health Assessment. [online] SDCEP. Available at: https://www.sdcep.org.uk/published-guidance/oral-health-assessment/.

Sheiham, A., 1992. The role of the dental team in promoting dental health and general health through oral health. International dental journal, 42(4), pp.223-228.

Sheiham, A., 2006. Dental caries affects body weight, growth and quality of life in pre-school children. British Dental Journal, 201(10), pp. 625–626.

Shulman, E. R., Howard, W. G., Sharps, G. and Wearden, S., 2011. The impact of a continuing education oral health program on providing services for young children by dentists, dental hygienists and dental assistants. American Dental Hygienists' Association, 85(3), pp. 220-228.

Tricco, A. C., Lillie, E., Zarin, W., O'Brien, K. K., Colquhoun, H., Levac, D., et al., 2018. PRISMA extension for scoping reviews (PRISMA-ScR): Checklist and explanation. Annals of Internal Medicine, 169(7), pp. 467–473. https://doi. org/10. 7326/M18-0850

Watt, R. G. and Sheiham, A., 2012. Integrating the common risk factor approach into a social determinants framework. Community Dentistry and Oral Epidemiology, 40(4), pp. 289–296.

www.who.int. (2024). Global strategy and action plan on oral health 2023–2030. [online] Available at: https://www.who.int/publications/i/item/9789240090538.

Appendix

Appendix A: Search Strategy

PCC Element	Keywords / Search Terms	MeSH Terms / Controlled Vocabulary	Synonyms / Variations
Population (P)	dental nurse* OR dental assistant* OR extended duty dental nurse*	"Dental Assistants"[MeSH]	dental auxiliary, oral health assistant, EDDN
Concept (C)	oral health promotion OR caries prevention OR health education OR fluoride varnish OR toothbrushing OR dietary counselling OR motivational interviewing	"Health Promotion"[MeSH], "Preventive Dentistry"[MeSH], "Fluorides, Topical"[MeSH], "Patient Education as Topic"[MeSH]	OHE, oral hygiene instruction, preventive care, anticipatory guidance, brushing programme

Context (C)	dental practice* OR general dental practice* OR primary dental care	"Dental Clinics"[MeSH], "General Practice"[MeSH]	general dentistry, primary care setting, NHS dental practice

Search String:

((((((dent* nurs*) OR (oral health nurs*) OR (dent* auxiliaries)) OR (dent* assistants)) AND ((((prevent*) OR (oral health promot*)) OR (fluoride varnish)) OR (oral hygiene instruction))) OR (dietary advice))) AND (((((dental caries) OR (early childhood caries)) OR (ECC)) OR (tooth decay)) OR (dental decay))) AND (general dental practice)

Appendix B – Search History

Date	Database / Source	Search Query / Keywords Used	Search Filters Applied	Results Retrieved
15 June 2025	**PubMed**	(((((dent* nurs*) OR (oral health nurs*) OR (dent* auxiliaries)) OR (dent* assistants)) AND ((((prevent*) OR (oral health promot*)) OR (fluoride varnish)) OR (oral hygiene instruction))) OR (dietary advice))) AND (((((dental caries) OR (early childhood caries)) OR (ECC)) OR (tooth decay)) OR (dental decay))) AND (general	English, Humans, 2000–2025	136

		dental practice)		
15 June 2025	**Embase**	Same as above	English, Humans, 2000–2025	36
15 June 2025	**Web of Science**	Same as above	English only, 2000–2025	7
15 June 2025	**Scopus**	Same as above	English only, 2000–2025	5
15 June 2025	**Google Scholar**	"Dental nurse" AND "oral health promotion" AND	English only, any year	1

		“children” AND “general dental practice”		
15 June 2025	**NHS Evidence**	“Dental nurse fluoride varnish children” / “oral health promotion by dental assistants in UK practices”	English only	1
15 June 2025	**WHO Website / Documents**	“Oral health promotion, dental nurse, children, general practice”	English only	0
	TOTAL RECORDS RETRIEVED			**186**
	Additional Notes	Search results were exported to EndNote 21, with 24 duplicates removed. After screening 162 articles, 14 full-text articles were		

		assessed, and 10 studies were included in the review. The PRISMA 2020 flow diagram is in Chapter 4.		

Appendix C- JBI Checklist Summary

Title of Study	**Author (Year)**	**Checklist Used**	**Overall Quality Judgment**
Barriers encountered during skill mix	Hatim & Kendall (2012)	Qualitative Research	Include an appropriate qualitative design
Communication skills for EDDNs	O'Keefe (2015)	Text and Opinion Papers	Include – informative expert perspective
Dental recurrence randomised trial	Pine et al. (2020)	Randomised Controlled Trials	Include – strong RCT design, some risk of bias
Effectiveness of oral health promotion interventions	Peerbhay et al. (2025)	Scoping Review	Included – Scoping review, no appraisal required
Effectiveness of preventive program after extractions	Gallagher et al. (2024)	Rapid Review	Included – Rapid review, no appraisal required

Evaluating Childsmile: Scotland's national program	Ross et al. (2023)	Analytical Cross-Sectional Studies	Include a robust national evaluation
Evaluation of EDDNs' experiences in Childsmile	Gnich et al. (2014)	Analytical Cross-Sectional Studies	Include – representative survey design
Getting help for children: improving access to dental care	Gehsan & Mijic (2019)	Quasi-Experimental Studies	Include a practical QI project
Impact of a continuing oral health program	Howard et al. (2017)	Quasi-Experimental Studies	Include – valid before-and-after analysis
Evaluation of Scotland's national oral health program	Kidd et al. (2020)	Analytical Cross-Sectional Studies	Include – strong Population trend data

Appendix D- Included articles

Title	Authors	Year	Population: Dental Nurses, Dental Auxiliaries, Dental Assistants	Concept: Oral Health Promotion - Activities:Toothbrushing and Oral Hygiene Advice, Fluoride Varnish Applications, Diet Counselling and Nutritional Advice, Oral Health Education, Behavioural Change Interventions	Context: General Dental Practice	Target group Children (0-18)	Overall Assessment (Must have Yes indicators f all three PC compoents
Barriers enc	Hatim E, Kend	Prim Dent	Yes	Yes	Yes	Yes	Included
Communica	O'Keefe E.	Prim Dent	Yes	Yes	Yes	Yes	Included
Dental RECI	Pine CM, Adai	J Dent Re	Yes	Yes	Yes	Yes	Included
Effectivene	Peerbhay F, M	PLoS One	Yes	Yes	Yes	Yes	Included
Effectivene	Kouassi SM, S	Communit	Yes	Yes	Yes	Yes	Included
Evaluating c	Ross AJ, Sher	Communit	Yes	Yes	Yes	Yes	Included
Evaluation c	Kidd JB, McM	BMJ Open	Yes	Yes	Yes	Yes	Included
Getting help	Gehshan S, Mi	J Calif De	Yes	Yes	Yes	Yes	Included
The impact	Shulman ER, I	J Dent Hy	Yes	Yes	Yes	Yes	Included
Extending d	Gnich W, Deas	BMC Oral	Yes	Yes	Yes	Yes	Included

Included Articles-10

Appendix E- Data Charting Table

Study	Country	Role of a Dental Nurse	Target Group	Intervention	Outcome
Hatim & Kendall (2012)	UK	EDDNs applied fluoride after CPD training	Children (0–18 yrs)	Fluoride varnish	Positive feedback; barriers due to cost & policy
O'Keefe (2015)	UK Scotland	EDDNs trained in communication and fluoride use	Deprived children	Fluoride varnish, communication support	No formal outcomes measured
Pine et al. (2020)	UK	Dental nurses delivered MI sessions to parents	5–7 yrs post-extraction	Motivational Interviewing	51% caries reduction (p=0.021)
Peerbhay et al. (2025)	Global	Nurses co-delivered oral health education	8–18 yrs	OHP with MI, brushing, fluoride	Mixed results; nurse-specific impact unclear
Kouassi et al. (2023)	UK	Nurses delivered fluoride & OHP post-extraction	0–19 yrs	Fluoride, education, MI	Improved oral health; the nurse's role is not isolated
Ross et al. (2023)	UK Scotland	Nurses delivered fluoride, brushing, and advice	0–12 yrs (focus: deprived)	Comprehensive OHP	Cost-effective; reduced caries

Kidd et al. (2023)	UK Scotland	Nurses supported fluoride & health advice	5-year-olds	Varnish, diet & brushing support	Lower carie in the high exposure group
Gehshan & Mijic (2011)	USA	Hygienists/ therapists led school prevention	0–18 yrs	Sealants, fluoride, and education	Improved access & care delive
Shulman et al. (2011)	USA	Hygienists/ assistants trained for ECC	0–3 yrs	ECC education, fluoride	↑knowledg & confidence 42% practice change
Gnich et al. (2015)	UK Scotland	EDDNs delivered fluoride & education	3–5 yrs	Fluoride, health sessions	94% varnish, strong role confidence

www.ingramcontent.com/pod-product-compliance
Lightning Source LLC
LaVergne TN
LVHW022112200926
848481LV00003B/1152
* 9 7 8 1 9 1 8 4 2 4 7 4 4 *